The Official Pocket Guide to

Diabetes Food Choices

6th Edition

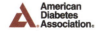

American
Diabetes
Association.

VP & Publisher, Professional Publications, Chris Kohler; *Director, Strategy & Editorial ,* John Clark; *Director, Book Operations,* Victor Van Beuren; *Director, Book Marketing,* Annette Reape; *Composition,* Jeska Horgan-Kobelski; *Printer,* Versa Press.

Printed in the United States of America

1 3 5 7 9 10 8 6 4 2

The suggestions and information contained in this publication are generally consistent with the *Standards of Care in Diabetes* and other policies of the American Diabetes Association, but they do not represent the policy or position of the Association or any of its boards or committees. Reasonable steps have been taken to ensure the accuracy of the information presented. However, the American Diabetes Association cannot ensure the safety or efficacy of any product or service described in this publication. Individuals are advised to consult a physician or other appropriate health care professional before undertaking any diet or exercise program or taking any medication referred to in this publication. Professionals must use and apply their own professional judgment, experience, and training and should not rely solely on the information contained in this publication before prescribing any diet, exercise, or medication. The American Diabetes Association—its officers, directors, employees, volunteers, and members—assumes no responsibility or liability for personal or other injury, loss, or damage that may result from the suggestions or information in this publication.

∞ The paper in this publication meets the requirements of the ANSI Standard Z39.48-1992 (permanence of paper).

ADA titles may be purchased for business or promotional use or for special sales. To purchase more than 50 copies of this book at a discount, or for custom editions of this book with your logo, contact the American Diabetes Association at booksales@diabetes.org.

American Diabetes Association
2451 Crystal Drive, Suite 900
Arlington, VA 22202

DOI: 10.2337/9781580408417

Library of Congress Control Number: 2025935906

CONTENTS

HEALTHY EATING

An Important Step in Taking Care of Your Diabetes

If you have diabetes, you do not need to eat special foods. The foods that are good for everyone are also good for you. This book can help you choose healthy foods in the right portion sizes to keep your blood glucose (blood sugar) within your target range.

A healthy eating plan:

- Includes a mix of foods each day: vegetables, fruits, whole grains, legumes (beans, lentils, and peas), low-fat and fat-free milk products, seafood, lean meats, poultry, plant-based protein foods, and nuts and seeds
- Limits foods that are high in sodium (salt), solid fats, and added sugars
- Helps you manage your blood glucose and meet your weight goals

A registered dietitian nutritionist (RDN) (referred to as dietitian in this guide) can help you learn how to take care of your diabetes. A registered dietitian nutritionist is a health professional who is an expert in nutrition care, education, and counseling. A certified diabetes care and education specialist (CDCES) is a health professional who has advanced training and is an expert in the care of people with diabetes (or prediabetes) specifically.

How Eating Affects Your Blood Glucose

Your body needs insulin (made by the pancreas) to use these nutrients correctly. When you eat foods, especially those that contain carbohydrates (carbs), they turn into glucose (a type of sugar). Glucose is the fuel that powers all the cells in your body. Insulin helps move glucose into your cells. When a person has diabetes, the pancreas does not make insulin or does not make enough insulin to get glucose into the body's cells.

Many people with type 2 diabetes or prediabetes also have insulin resistance. When you have insulin resistance, your body cannot use insulin properly. At first, your pancreas makes extra insulin to make up for this. But, over time, your pancreas is not able to keep up and cannot make enough insulin to keep the blood glucose in a healthy range. The good news is that cutting calories, being active, and losing weight can reduce your insulin resistance. For people with prediabetes, these lifestyle changes can also reduce your risk for heart disease and prevent or delay type 2 diabetes.

To keep your blood glucose within your target range, try to eat about the same amount of food, especially carbs, around the same times each day. Skipping meals may lead to low blood glucose if you use insulin or certain glucose-lowering medications. However, if you inject insulin or use an insulin pump to manage your blood glucose, you have more freedom to vary what you eat at each meal.

No matter how you manage your diabetes, plan to spread your meals and snacks throughout the day. Your dietitian can help you decide the timing and size of meals and snacks that are right for you.

Healthy Eating, Physical Activity, and Your Weight

The foods you eat give you energy (or calories). Your body uses these calories to help you breathe, sit, walk, or move (physical activity). If you eat the amount of calories that your body uses for daily activity on most days, your weight should stay about the same. You will gain weight if you eat more calories than your body uses on most days. When you eat fewer calories than your body uses for energy, you lose weight because your body must burn stored calories. If you are at a healthy weight, you can stay at that weight by eating the right amount of food for your needs along with physical activity. Your diabetes team can help you plan calorie and physical activity goals that are realistic.

How to Be More Active

Physical activity may lower overall blood glucose and reduce insulin resistance, blood pressure, and cholesterol levels. Regular physical activity may also help you manage your weight.

Here are some tips to help be more active:

- Choose an activity you enjoy. Many people enjoy walking because it is easy to do and is free.

- Start with a daily goal of 5 to 10 minutes of activity, such as walking at a pace and distance that feels comfortable. Work up to at least 30 minutes a day, 5 times a week. Short amounts of activity count, such as 3 walks that are 10 minutes long.

- Include strength training for muscles at least 2 times a week in your activity plan.

- Wear comfortable shoes with proper fit and good traction.

- Move more in your everyday activities. Take the stairs instead of the elevator. Park your car farther away from work or the store. Walk to the next bus or subway stop to get a few more steps in.

- Put extra effort into housework and chores, such as washing windows, scrubbing floors, vacuuming, and raking the yard.

- Have backup plans for bad weather. Walk at a mall or warehouse store or find indoor activities you enjoy, such as walking on a treadmill, or find a workout program online, on your TV, or through an app (such as on your smartphone or tablet).

If you have concerns about how to get started with a physical activity program, talk with your healthcare provider.

Planning Healthy Meals

An Eating Plan (see page 92) helps you choose healthy meals for each day of the week. You and your RDN or CDCES will discuss your plan choices together. This eating plan is your guide to picking the number of choices from three of the food categories listed in this booklet that is right for you at each meal and snack. In this plan, the number of choices from each food category is based on your calorie and nutrient needs, your lifestyle, your usual schedule of eating, and your diabetes management plan. Planning healthy meals will help you:

- Keep your blood glucose within your target range
- Reach and maintain a healthy weight
- Manage blood cholesterol and blood lipid (fat) levels
- Control your blood pressure

How Are these Recommendations Developed?

The Standards of Care in Diabetes is published by the American Diabetes Association (ADA). It is a set of diabetes-management guidelines used by healthcare professionals based on the latest scientific research and clinical trials. Every 5 years, a group of external experts comes together for an in-depth review of the nutrition aspect of the guidelines. This report is called the Nutrition Consensus.

The Nutrition Consensus is the foundation for the ADA's nutrition recommendations. The goal is to determine nutrition methods that work toward improving or maintaining glycemic targets, achieving weight management goals, and improving risk factors for co-occurring conditions based upon a person's individual needs.

The current Consensus outlines seven key meal patterns that are recognized to improve diabetes management. It is up to the person with diabetes to work with their healthcare team to decide which pattern works best for their personal needs.

How Is a Meal Pattern Different from a Diet, and Which Pattern Is Best for Diabetes?

Healthcare professionals prefer to use terms like "meal pattern" insead of "diet" to better represent when, what, and how much we eat on a daily basis. Diet is a tricky word. It has a lot of connotations and can carry emotional baggage for some people. And a diet is usually more of a short-term approach than a long-term lifestyle change. Meal patterns tend to offer a more sustainable approach. An eating plan provides the details that help you follow the pattern you like. This makes it easier to know what to shop for, cook, or choose when eating out.

So the answer to the question is that there isn't a "best" meal pattern—there's no scientific evidence that supports a one-size-fits-all pattern for the prevention or management of diabetes. There are millions of people living with diabetes, and when you think about their cultural backgrounds, personal preferences, co-occurring conditions, and socioeconomic situations, you'll probably understand why there is no "one simple trick" to nutrition that works for everyone.

This is why the ADA focuses on several meal patterns that are scientifically proven to be effective in diabetes management. These meal patterns are meant to be sustainable, long-term ways of eating. While diets may cause you to lose weight quickly at first, it's more important to focus on food choices that you enjoy and can be successfully integrated into your lifestyle.

Suggested Meal Pattern for Diabetes Management

Diabetes management requires a lifestyle change. When considering what meal pattern will work best for you, consider the types of foods you like to eat, the time you have to prepare food, your budget, and even your family's dietary needs. Consult with your healthcare team about which of the following meal patterns might work well for you based on your particular tastes, health needs, and goals.

Mediterranean-Style Meal Pattern

This pattern is great for people who are looking to reduce their risk of diabetes, seeking to reduce their A1C, lower their triglycerides, or reduce their risk of cardiovascular events.

Mediterranean-Style meal pattern highlights:

- Plant-based foods (vegetables, beans, nuts and seeds, fruits, and whole grains)
- Fish and other seafood
- Olive oil as the principal source of dietary fat
- Dairy products (mainly yogurt and cheese) in low to moderate amounts
- Typically, fewer than four eggs/week
- Red meat in low frequency and amounts
- Wine in low to moderate amounts
- Concentrated sugars or honey rarely

Vegetarian or Vegan Meal Patterns

For people who are looking to reduce their risk of diabetes, seeking to reduce their A1C, achieve weight loss, or reduce their LDL and non-HDL cholesterol values, one of these patterns would be a good choice.

Vegetarian or Vegan meal pattern highlights:

- Meal pattern exclusively using plant-based foods, excluding all animal-based products (**vegan**), or a pattern that excludes meats, seafood, or poultry but includes eggs and/or dairy products (**vegetarian**).

Low-Fat Meal Pattern

The Low-Fat meal pattern is excellent for people who are looking to reduce their risk of diabetes or seeking to achieve weight loss.

Low-fat meal pattern highlights:
- Vegetables
- Fruits
- Starches (e.g., breads/crackers, pasta, whole grains, starchy vegetables)
- Lean protein sources (including beans)
- Low-fat dairy products

In this review of the nutrition consensus, low fat was defined as total fat intake less than 30% of total calories, with saturated fat intake of less than 10%.

Very Low-Fat Meal Pattern

For people who are looking to achieve weight loss or reduce their blood pressure, this meal pattern may be a good choice.

Very low-fat meal pattern highlights:
- Fiber-rich vegetables
- Beans
- Fruits
- Whole grains
- Non-fat dairy
- Fish
- Egg whites

This pattern comprises 70–77% carbohydrate (including 30–60 g fiber) and less than 10% total calories from fat.

Low-Carbohydrate Meal Pattern

This pattern is good for people who are looking to reduce their A1C, achieve weight loss, lower their blood pressure, lower triglycerides, or increase HDL cholesterol.

Low carb meal pattern highlights:
- Non-starchy vegetables low in carbohydrates
- Healthy fats
- Protein in the form of meat, poultry, fish, shellfish, eggs, cheese, nuts, and seeds
- Quality carbohydrates are included but limited.

In this review, a low-carbohydrate eating pattern is defined as reducing carbohydrates to 26–45% of total calories.

Very Low-Carbohydrate Meal Pattern

For people who are looking to reduce their A1C, achieve weight loss, lower their blood pressure, lower triglycerides, or increase HDL cholesterol, this pattern may well be a good choice.

The Very Low-Carbohydrate meal pattern is similar to the low-carbohydrate pattern but limits carbohydrate-containing foods even further. Meals typically contain more than half of calories from fat. This pattern often has a goal of 20–50 g of non-fiber carbohydrate per day. In this review, a very low-carbohydrate eating pattern is defined as reducing carbohydrate to less than 26% of total calories.

Dietary Approaches to Stop Hypertension (DASH) Meal Pattern

This pattern is helpful for people who are looking to reduce their risk of diabetes, seeking to achieve weight loss, or lower their blood pressure.

DASH meal pattern highlights:
- Vegetables
- Fruits
- Low-fat dairy products
- Whole grains
- Poultry
- Fish
- Nuts
- Reduced saturated fat, red meat, sweets, and sugar-containing beverages.
- May also be reduced in sodium.

Using the Diabetes Plate Method with Meal Patterns

The Diabetes Plate Method (see page 93) can be a framework for all meal patterns. The Plate Method is basically a simple representation of the Low-Carbohydrate Meal Pattern. By using the specific strategies outlined in each of the meal patterns, the Diabetes Plate Method can be used to help imagine how each pattern can be turned into breakfast, lunch, or dinner.

Whether you live with prediabetes, type 1 or type 2 diabetes, have co-occurring considerations like heart or kidney-disease, or have gestational diabetes, informed food choices are essential to managing your health. Work with your healthcare team to find the best meal pattern and management strategies that work for you. If you respond best to carbohydrate counting or limit certain foods that have more of an impact on your own blood glucose, this is the kind of knowledge you pick up to help you master your own diabetes management. Find what works best for you!

Other Factors Impacting Your Diabetes Management

While healthy eating is a crucial aspect of managing your blood glucose (blood sugar), there are many other factors to consider as well. It is important to understand how these other elements of daily living impact you.

Diabetes Management Coping The daily challenges of managing your diabetes can cause stress and influence how you feel about your overall well-being. When your coping skills are challenged, it can be more difficult to make healthy eating choices. Understanding the impact of diabetes on your mental health can help you embrace the skills needed to deal with daily decision making, stress, and barriers to healthy eating.

Physical Activity Physical activity is important to your overall health for a number of reasons, especially when you are living with diabetes. By making healthy food choices, you fuel your body with the right kinds of energy needed to help you move, exercise, and thrive.

Medications Understanding how your medications work in combination with your meal timing and food choices helps you better manage your diabetes and prevent complications.

Monitoring Keeping track of your daily activities, eating, and stress levels provides feedback on how your lifestyle influences your blood glucose levels. Writing this information down helps you see patterns that suggest changes you can make to meet your goals.

Health Risks Knowing how to prevent, detect, and treat both immediate and long-term risks are important to preventing diabetes complications. Healthy eating helps to prevent hypoglycemia (low blood glucose) or hyperglycemia (high blood glucose). Over time, reducing these daily lows and highs can reduce your chances of developing diabetes complications, or help you better manage and limit their progression.

Biology Every body is different. Understanding how yours responds to the changes you will probably face in your diabetes journey helps you find the therapies and strategies that contribute to your health goals. Healthy eating, physical activity, medication, and other parts of daily life with diabetes may need to be modified from time to time to better support your successful diabetes management.

To help you gain the knowledge, skills, and confidence to thrive with diabetes, use the following link to find a diabetes education program: *diabetes.org/tools-resources/diabetes-education-programs.* Highly trained and specialized healthcare providers, such as diabetes care and education specialists, are ready to work closely with you to find practical solutions that fit your personal needs.

The Food Lists

The food lists in this booklet group foods together that have about the same amount of carbohydrates (carbs), protein, fat, and calories. The term **choice** is used to describe a certain quantity of food within a group of similar foods.

The lists are grouped into 3 main types:

1. **Carbohydrates** include the **Starch** list (breads, cereals, grains, starchy vegetables, crackers, beans, peas, and lentils), **Fruits** list, and **Milk and Milk Substitutes** list. These lists are similar because each choice contains about 12 to 15 grams of carbs in the serving size listed. It also includes the **Nonstarchy Vegetables** list (such as green beans, tomatoes, and carrots), which contain about 5 grams of carbs for each choice.

2. **Proteins** include lists for **Lean Protein, Medium-Fat Protein, High-Fat Protein,** and **Plant-Based Protein.** Meat, poultry, and fish contain no carbs and varying amounts of fat, while plant-based protein foods often contain some carbs.

3. **Fats** include lists for the healthier **Unsaturated Fats** and for less healthy **Saturated Fats.** These choices contain only fat and calories.

Other types of foods that you may eat are included in the **Sweets, Desserts, and Other Carbohydrates** list and **Combination Foods** list (such as casseroles). These lists have foods that have different amounts of carbs, protein, fat, and calories. Foods eaten between meals and extras, such as some fat-free and reduced-fat foods, condiments, drinks, and seasonings, can be found on the **Snacks and**

Extras list. Drinks on the **Alcohol** list contain calories, and some contain carbs.

The following chart shows the amount of nutrients in 1 choice from each list.

FOOD LIST	CARBS (GRAMS)	PROTEIN (GRAMS)	FAT (GRAMS)	CALORIES
Carbohydrates				
Starch: breads; cereals; grains and pasta; starchy vegetables; crackers and snacks; beans, peas, and lentils	15	3	1	80
Fruits	15	—	—	60
Milk and Milk Substitutes				
fat-free, low-fat, 1%	12	8	0–3	100
reduced-fat, 2%	12	8	5	120
whole	12	8	8	160
Nonstarchy Vegetables	5	2	—	25
Sweets, Desserts, and Other Carbohydrates	15	varies	varies	varies

FOOD LIST	CARBS (GRAMS)	PROTEIN (GRAMS)	FAT (GRAMS)	CALORIES
Proteins				
Lean	–	7	2	45
Medium-Fat	–	7	5	75
High-Fat	–	7	8	100
Plant-Based	varies	7	varies	varies
Fats	–	–	5	45
	varies	–	–	100

The following symbols are used throughout this booklet to let you know which foods are good sources of fiber, which have extra or added fat, and which are high in sodium.

🟠 **Good source of fiber** = More than 3 grams of dietary fiber per choice.

🔺 or 🔺 **Added fat** = A food with 1 or 2 extra fat choices.

🟠 **High in sodium** = 480 milligrams or more of sodium per choice. (For foods listed as a main dish/meal on the **Combination Foods** list only, the 🟠 represents more than 600 milligrams of sodium per choice.)

Cut Back on Salt and Solid Fats

Eating less salt (sodium) and solid (saturated and *trans*) fat is good for everyone, not just people with diabetes. High blood pressure can get worse if you eat too much sodium (from salt and salty foods). Reducing the amount and type of fat you eat may help you lower your risk of heart disease.

- When possible, use less salt in cooking and at the table. Snack foods, processed foods, canned soups, frozen meals and desserts, and restaurant food all tend to be high in sodium.

- Limit your choices of foods with saturated fat, such as higher-fat meats, butter, whole-milk dairy products, and tropical oils (coconut and palm oils).

Getting Started

Your dietitian will help you learn how to use the food lists in this booklet to improve your eating and physical activity habits. Together, you can adjust your eating plan when your lifestyle or activity levels change. For example, you can change your eating plan to fit your work, school, vacation, or travel schedule.

Your dietitian can also help you learn when to check your blood glucose and what the numbers mean. By checking your blood glucose, you learn how different foods affect your blood glucose, and you can often figure out when you need to make changes in your eating plan or diabetes self-care plan. As you take on healthy eating habits and learn how to manage your blood glucose, you will feel better, too.

Portion Sizes

 = 1 CUP

 = 1 OZ MEAT OR CHEESE

 = 1 TBSP

 = 1 TSP

 = 1 INCH

 = 1-2 OZ NUTS OR PRETZELS

 = 3 OZ MEAT, FISH, OR POULTRY

Portion size is an important part of meal planning. Try using the following comparisons to help measure portion sizes:

- 1 cup is about the size of an average fist.
- 1 ounce of cheese or cooked meat, poultry, or fish is about the size of the base of a thumb.
- 3 ounces of cooked meat, poultry, or fish is about the size of a woman's palm. The palm of a man's hand is about the size of 4 to 6 ounces of cooked meat, poultry, or fish.
- 1 tablespoon is about the size of a thumb.
- 1 teaspoon is about the size of a fingertip.

STARCH

Starches include bread, cereal, grains (including pasta and rice), starchy vegetables (such as green peas, corn, and potatoes), legumes (refried beans, black beans, split peas, black-eyed peas, and lentils), crackers, and snacks.

In general, 1 starch choice is:

- ½ cup of cooked cereal, grain, or starchy vegetable
- ⅓ cup of cooked rice or pasta
- 1 ounce of a bread product, such as 1 slice of bread
- ¾ to 1 ounce of crackers or grain-based snack foods

Eating Plan Tips

- For health benefits, choose whole grains for at least ½ of your servings of grains each day (see page 24 for more about whole grains).
- Choose starches made with little or no added fat.
- Starchy vegetables, baked goods, and grains that are prepared with fat count as 1 starch choice and 1 to 2 fat choices.
- For many starchy foods (bagels, muffins, dinner rolls, buns), 1 ounce equals 1 serving. Because of their large size, these foods often have more carbs and calories than you might think. For example, a large bagel may weigh 4 ounces and equal 4 starch choices.
- For information about fiber and other nutrients in grain foods, read the Nutrition Facts panel on the food label.

Gluten-Free Foods

Gluten is a protein in wheat, rye, and barley. If you have a gluten allergy or celiac disease and cannot eat foods that contain gluten, be sure to read food labels carefully.

- Foods labeled gluten-free can be part of your diabetes eating plan.

- For foods not labeled gluten-free, read the ingredients list. If you must follow a gluten-free eating plan, do not eat foods that list wheat, barley, rye, malt, brewer's yeast, or regular oats.

- When following a gluten-free eating plan, you can still eat many starch foods, including:
  - Baked goods, cereal, pasta, and other foods made with naturally gluten-free grains, such as brown rice or quinoa instead of wheat, rye, or barley.
  - Starchy vegetables, such as corn and potatoes.
  - Legumes, such as beans, peas, and lentils.

Bread

FOOD	SERVING SIZE
Bagel	¼ large bagel (1 oz)
Biscuit ⚠	1 biscuit (2½ inches across)
Breads, loaf-type	
whole wheat, whole grain, pumpernickel, rye, white, sourdough, French, Italian, unfrosted raisin, or cinnamon	1 slice (1 oz)
gluten-free	1 slice (1 oz)
reduced-calorie, light ✓	2 slices (1½ oz)
Breads, flat-type (flatbreads)	
chapati	1 oz
ciabatta	1 oz
Indian fry bread ⚠	⅙ piece (1 oz)
naan	3¼-inch square (1 oz)
pita	½ pita (6 inches across)
roti	1 oz
sandwich flat buns, whole wheat ✓	1 bun, including top and bottom (1½ oz)
taco shell ⚠	2 taco shells (5 inches across)
tortilla, corn	1 small tortilla (6 inches across)
tortilla, flour (white or whole wheat)	1 small tortilla (6 inches across) or ⅓ large tortilla (10 inches across)
Cornbread	1¾-inch cube (1½ oz)
English muffin	½ muffin
Hot dog bun or hamburger bun	½ bun (¾ oz)

Bread, continued

FOOD	SERVING SIZE
Pancake	1 pancake (4 inches across, ¼-inch thick)
Roll, plain	1 small roll (1 oz)
Stuffing, bread ⚠	⅓ cup
Waffle	1 waffle (4-inch square or 4 inches across)

⚠ count as 1 starch choice + 1 fat choice (1 starch choice plus 5 grams of fat)

Cereals

FOOD	SERVING SIZE
Bran cereal (twigs, buds, or flakes) ✓	½ cup
Cooked cereals (oats, oatmeal)	½ cup
Granola cereal	¼ cup
Grits, cooked	½ cup
Muesli	¼ cup
Puffed cereal	1½ cups
Shredded wheat, plain	½ cup
Sugar-coated cereal	½ cup
Unsweetened, ready-to-eat cereal	¾ cup

Grains (Including Pasta and Rice)

Unless otherwise indicated, serving sizes listed are for cooked grains.

FOOD	SERVING SIZE
Amaranth	⅓ cup
Barley	⅓ cup
Bran, dry	
oat ✅	¼ cup
wheat ✅	½ cup
Buckwheat	½ cup
Bulgur ✅	½ cup
Couscous	⅓ cup
Farro	½ cup
Kamut	½ cup
Kasha	½ cup
Millet	⅓ cup
Pasta, white, whole wheat, multigrain, gluten-free (all shapes and sizes)	⅓ cup
Quinoa, all colors	⅓ cup
Rice, white, brown, and other colors and types	⅓ cup
Sorghum	⅓ cup
Tabbouleh (tabouli), prepared	½ cup
Wheat germ, dry	3 Tbsp
Wild rice	½ cup

Whole Grains

Whole grains and whole-grain foods contain all parts of the grain seed of a plant. Whole grains and foods made with whole grains give you fiber, vitamins, and minerals. Here are some tips for choosing more whole grains:

- Read labels and look for "whole grain" or "whole wheat" on the front of a package. In the ingredient list, look for products with the word "whole" in front of the first ingredient.

- Try to include more foods made with whole grains, such as whole-wheat bread, whole-wheat pasta, whole-grain crackers, whole-grain tortillas, and pita bread.

- Some whole grains can be added to other foods, such as stews, soups, or salads, or they can be enjoyed on their own. Examples include whole oats/oatmeal, whole-grain cornmeal, popcorn, buckwheat, whole-grain barley, brown rice, wild rice, bulgur, millet, quinoa, and sorghum.

Starchy Vegetables

All of the serving sizes for starchy vegetables on this list are for cooked vegetables.

FOOD	SERVING SIZE
Breadfruit	¼ cup
Cassava or dasheen	⅓ cup
Corn, kernel	½ cup
Corn on the cob	3⅞- to 4½-inch piece (½ large)
Hominy ✅	¾ cup
Mixed vegetables with corn or peas ✅	1 cup
Marinara, pasta, or spaghetti sauce	½ cup
Parsnips ✅	½ cup
Peas, green ✅	½ cup
Plantain	⅓ cup
Potato	
baked with skin	¼ large potato (3 oz)
boiled, all kinds	½ cup or ½ medium potato (3 oz)
hash browns ⚠️	½ cup
mashed, with milk and fat ⚠️	½ cup
French fried (oven-baked)*	1 cup (2 oz)
Pumpkin purée, canned, no sugar added ✅	¾ cup
Squash, winter (acorn, butternut) ✅	1 cup
Succotash ✅	½ cup
Yam or sweet potato, plain	½ cup (3½ oz)

Crackers and Snacks

Please note, some snacks are high in fat. Always check food labels.

FOOD	SERVING SIZE
Crackers	
animal	8 crackers
crispbread ✅	2 to 5 pieces (¾ oz)
graham, 2½-inch square	3 squares
nut and rice	10 crackers
oyster	20 crackers
round, butter-type ⚠️	6 crackers
saltine-type	6 crackers
sandwich-style, cheese or peanut butter filling ⚠️	3 crackers
whole-wheat, baked	5 regular 1½-inch squares or 10 thins (¾ oz)
Granola or snack bar	1 bar (¾ oz)
Matzoth (matzo), all shapes and sizes	¾ oz
Melba toast	4 pieces (each about 2 by 4 inches)
Popcorn	
no fat added ✅	3 cups
with butter added ⚠️	3 cups
Pretzels	¾ oz
Rice cakes	2 cakes (4 inches across)

Crackers and Snacks, continued

FOOD	SERVING SIZE
Snack chips	
baked (potato, pita)	about 8 chips (¾ oz)
regular (tortilla, potato) ⚠️	about 13 chips (1 oz)

NOTE: For other snacks, see the Snacks and Extras list, pages 74–76, and the Sweets, Desserts, and Other Carbohydrates list, pages 66–73.

Beans, Peas, and Lentils

The choices on this list count as 1 starch choice + 1 lean protein choice.

FOOD	SERVING SIZE
Baked beans, canned ✅	⅓ cup
Beans (black, garbanzo, kidney, lima, navy, pinto, white), cooked or canned, drained and rinsed ✅	½ cup
Lentils (any color), cooked ✅	½ cup
Peas (black-eyed and split), cooked or canned, drained and rinsed ✅	½ cup
Refried beans, canned ✅ 🥄	½ cup

NOTE: Beans, lentils, and peas are also found on the Protein list, pages 48–41.

Sodium in Canned Foods

Canned vegetables, such as beans, lentils, and peas, can be high in sodium (salt). Draining and rinsing them reduces the sodium content by about 40%.

FRUITS

Fresh, frozen, canned, and dried fruit and fruit juices are on this list.

In general, 1 fruit choice is:

- ½ cup of unsweetened canned or frozen fruit
- 1 small fresh fruit (about 2½ inches in diameter)
- ½ cup (4 fluid ounces) of unsweetened fruit juice (100% juice)
- 2 tablespoons of dried fruit

Eating Plan Tips

- Fresh and frozen fruit are good sources of fiber. Fruit juice contains very little fiber and can raise your blood glucose very fast. Choose whole fruit instead of juice more often.

- Fruit smoothies may contain many servings of fruit. If you can, make your own. If you buy a fruit smoothie, ask to find out if they add sugar, syrup, or sweetened fruit juices.

- Some fruits on the list are measured by weight. The weights listed include skin, core, seeds, and rind. Use a food scale to weigh fresh fruits to figure out how many choices you are eating.

- Read the Nutrition Facts on food labels of packaged fruits and juices. If 1 serving has more than 15 grams of carbs, you may need to adjust the size of the serving to fit with the choices in your eating plan.

- Serving sizes for canned fruits on the **Fruits** list are for the fruit and a small amount (1 to 2 tablespoons) of juice (not syrup).

- Food labels for fruits and fruit juices may contain the words "no sugar added" or "unsweetened." This means that no sugar—other than the sugar from the fruit itself—has been added. Note that these will still contain carbs.

- Fruit canned in extra-light syrup has the same amount of carbs per serving as canned fruit labeled "no sugar added" or "juice pack." All canned fruits on the **Fruits** list are based on 1 of these 3 types of packs. Avoid fruit canned in heavy syrup.

Fruits

The weight listed includes skin, core, seeds, and rind.

FOOD	SERVING SIZE
Apple, unpeeled	1 small apple (4 oz)
Apples, dried	4 rings
Applesauce, unsweetened	½ cup
Apricots	
canned	½ cup
dried	8 apricot halves
fresh	4 apricots (5½ oz total)
Asian pear, apple pear	1 medium Asian pear (4 oz)

FOOD	SERVING SIZE
Banana	1 extra-small banana, or about 4-inch-long piece (4 oz)
Blackberries ✅	1 cup
Blueberries	¾ cup
Cantaloupe	1 cup diced
Cherries	
sweet, canned	½ cup
sweet, fresh	12 cherries (3½ oz)
Clementine, mandarin orange	2 small (2½ oz each)
Dates	3 small (deglet noor) dates or 1 large (medjool) date
Dried fruits (blueberries, cherries, cranberries, mixed fruit, raisins)	2 Tbsp
Figs	
dried	3 small figs
fresh ✅	1½ large or 2 medium figs (3½ oz total)
Fruit cocktail	½ cup
Grapefruit	
fresh	½ large grapefruit (5½ oz)
sections, canned	¾ cup

Fruits, continued

FOOD	SERVING SIZE
Grapes	17 small grapes (3 oz)
Guava ✓	2 small guava (2½ oz)
Honeydew melon	1 cup diced
Huckleberries, fresh	1 cup
Kiwi	½ cup sliced
Kumquat	5 pieces (size of a large olive)
Loquat	¾ cup cubed
Mandarin oranges, canned	¾ cup
Mango	½ small mango (5½ oz) or ½ cup
Nectarine	1 medium nectarine (5½ oz)
Orange ✓	1 medium orange (6½ oz)
Papaya	½ papaya (8 oz) or 1 cup cubed
Passion fruit	½ cup
Peaches	
canned	½ cup
fresh	1 medium peach (6 oz)
Pears	
canned	½ cup
fresh ✓	½ large pear (4 oz)

FOOD	SERVING SIZE
Pineapple	
canned	½ cup
fresh	¾ cup
Plantain, extra-ripe (black), raw	¼ plantain (2¼ oz)
Plums	
canned	½ cup
dried (prunes)	3
fresh	2 small plums (5 oz total)
Pomegranate seeds (arils)	½ cup
Raspberries ✅	1 cup
Strawberries ✅	1¼ cups whole berries
Tamarillo	1 cup
Tangerine	1 large tangerine (6 oz)
Watermelon	1¼ cups diced

Fruit Juice

FOOD	SERVING SIZE
Apple juice/cider	½ cup (4 fl oz)
Fruit juice blends, 100% juice	⅓ cup (2.7 fl oz)
Grape juice	⅓ cup (2.7 fl oz)
Grapefruit juice	½ cup (4 fl oz)
Orange juice	½ cup (4 fl oz)
Pineapple juice	½ cup (4 fl oz)
Pomegranate juice	½ cup (4 fl oz)
Prune juice	⅓ cup (2.7 fl oz)

MILK AND MILK SUBSTITUTES

Milk, milk products, and milk substitutes are included on this list. In general, 1 milk choice is about 1 cup of milk or plain yogurt.

Other types of milk products are found on other lists:

- Cheeses are on the **Protein** list, and butter, cream, and coffee creamers are on the **Fats** list because these foods all have very few carbs.

- Ice cream and frozen yogurt are on the **Sweets, Desserts, and Other Carbohydrates** list.

Eating Plan Tips

- Milk and yogurt are good sources of calcium and protein. Be aware that grain-based or nut-based milks may be lower in calcium, protein, and other nutrients. Look for those fortified in calcium and vitamin D with a similar amount of protein as milk.

- Greek yogurt often contains more protein and fewer carbs than other types of yogurt.

- Milk and yogurt types that are higher in fat (those made from 2% or whole milk) have more saturated fat, cholesterol, and calories than low-fat or fat-free milk and yogurt.

- Health professionals suggest that adults and children older than 2 years choose lower-fat milk and milk products, such as fat-free (skim) or low-fat (1%) milk, or low-fat or nonfat yogurt.

- Remember that 1 cup = 8 fluid ounces or ½ pint. Most single-serve yogurt packs are between 4 and 6 ounces, which is about ½ to ¾ cup.

One milk choice has 12 grams of carbs and 8 grams of protein, and:

- One fat-free (skim) or low-fat (1%) milk choice also has 0 to 3 grams of fat and 100 calories per serving.

- One reduced-fat (2%) milk choice also has 5 grams of fat and 120 calories per serving.

- One whole-milk choice also has 8 grams of fat and 160 calories per serving.

Some milk foods and milk substitutes contain mostly carbs and fats:

- One carb choice has 15 grams of carbs and about 70 calories.

- One fat choice has 5 grams of fat and 45 calories.

Milk, Yogurt, and Milk Substitutes

FOOD	SERVING SIZE	CHOICES PER SERVING
Fat-free (skim) or low-fat (1%) milk		
milk, buttermilk, acidophilus milk, lactose-free milk	1 cup (8 fl oz)	1 fat-free milk
evaporated milk	½ cup (4 fl oz)	1 fat-free milk
yogurt, plain or Greek; may be flavored with a sugar substitute	⅔ cup (6 oz)	1 fat-free milk
yogurt with fruit, low-fat	⅔ cup (6 oz)	1 fat-free milk + 1 carb
chocolate milk	1 cup (8 fl oz)	1 fat-free milk + 1 carb
Reduced-fat (2%) milk		
milk, acidophilus milk, kefir, lactose-free milk	1 cup (8 fl oz)	1 reduced-fat milk
yogurt, plain	⅔ cup (6 oz)	1 reduced-fat milk
Whole milk		
milk, buttermilk, goat's milk	1 cup (8 fl oz)	1 whole milk
evaporated milk	½ cup (4 fl oz)	1 whole milk
yogurt, plain	1 cup (8 oz)	1 whole milk
chocolate milk	1 cup (8 fl oz)	1 whole milk + 1 carb

FOOD	SERVING SIZE	CHOICES PER SERVING
Eggnog		
fat-free	⅓ cup (2.7 fl oz)	1 carb
low-fat	⅓ cup (2.7 fl oz)	1 carb + ½ fat
whole milk	⅓ cup (2.7 fl oz)	1 carb + 1 fat
Rice milk		
plain, fat-free	1 cup (8 fl oz)	1 carb
flavored, low-fat	1 cup (8 fl oz)	2 carbs
Soy milk		
light or low-fat, plain	1 cup (8 fl oz)	½ carb + ½ fat
regular, plain	1 cup (8 fl oz)	1 carb + 1 fat
Almond milk		
plain	1 cup (8 fl oz)	½ carb + ½ fat
flavored	1 cup (8 fl oz)	1 carb + ½ fat
Coconut milk, flavored	1 cup (8 fl oz)	1 carb + 1 fat
Nondairy yogurt	1 cup (8 oz)	1 carb + 2 fats

NONSTARCHY VEGETABLES

Nonstarchy vegetables have fewer carbs and calories compared to starchy vegetables (such as potatoes, corn, and peas), and many also provide fiber. A nonstarchy vegetable choice is:

- ½ cup of cooked vegetables
- 1 cup of raw vegetables
- 3 cups of salad or leafy greens
- ½ cup (4 fluid ounces) vegetable juice

Eating Plan Tips

- Set a goal to eat at least 2 or 3 nonstarchy vegetable choices each day. Brightly colored, nonstarchy vegetables—such as dark-green, red, orange, and yellow vegetables—are packed with nutrients like vitamins A and C. Examples include broccoli, kale, beets, carrots, squash, and peppers.

- Potassium is a nutrient that helps your heart and can lower your blood pressure. All fruits and vegetables have some potassium. Good sources include tomatoes, spinach, mushrooms, Brussels sprouts, and carrots. If you have kidney disease and diabetes, talk to your dietitian about how much potassium is right for you.

- Fresh, plain vegetables have no added salt. When choosing canned or frozen vegetables, read food labels and look for low-sodium or no-salt-added varieties. If these are not available, you can drain and rinse canned vegetables to reduce the salt (sodium).

- Some canned and frozen vegetables also contain added fats and sauces, which can add calories and carbs as well as sodium. Be sure to check the Nutrition Facts label.

- The tomato sauce on this list is different from spaghetti/pasta sauce, which is on the **Starchy Vegetables** list because jars of sauce often have added sugar.

How to Eat More Vegetables

Try these ideas to help make it easy to enjoy more nonstarchy vegetables:

- Wash and cut up raw vegetables, like carrots, cucumber, bell peppers, celery, jicama, broccoli, and cauliflower, so that they are ready to use for meals and snacks.

- You can also buy precut fresh vegetables and ready-to-eat salad or leafy greens.

- Save time and buy bagged salad kits. Avoid using too much dressing and extra toppings, such as croutons and bacon bits, which often come with bagged salads.

- Add chopped (fresh, frozen, or canned) vegetables to anything you make, including rice, pasta, soups, casseroles, baked potatoes, sandwiches, scrambled eggs, or omelets.

- Challenge yourself to eat 3 (or more!) different colors of vegetables each day. Different colors help different parts of your body.

- Try new recipes like zucchini noodles, cauliflower rice, kale chips, roasted green beans, lettuce or collard green wraps, or baked turnip fries. Find fun new ways to enjoy your veggies.

- Store vegetables in the front and center of your refrigerator instead of hidden in the produce drawer. If you see them, you are more likely to eat them!

Nonstarchy Vegetables

Amaranth/Chinese spinach

Artichoke and artichoke hearts (packed in water)

Asparagus

Baby corn ✅

Bamboo shoots

Bean sprouts (alfalfa, mung, soybean)

Beets

Bok choy

Broccoli and Chinese broccoli, broccolini

Brussels sprouts ✅

Cabbage (green, purple, Chinese/Napa)

Carrots ✅

Cauliflower

Celery

Chayote ✅

Cucumber

Daikon

Eggplant and Chinese eggplant

Fennel

Gourds (bitter melon, bottle, luffa, snake, white)

Green beans and wax beans

Green onions, scallions, and chives

Greens (collard, mustard, turnip)

Nonstarchy Vegetables, continued

Hearts of palm
Jicama ✅
Kale
Kimchi 🔶
Kohlrabi
Leeks
Mushrooms, all kinds, fresh
Nopales
Okra
Onions and shallots
Pea pods
Pea shoots/pea vines
Peppers (bell, chile, and other kinds)
Radishes
Rutabaga
Salad or leafy greens (arugula, chicory, endive, escarole, lettuce, radicchio, romaine, and watercress)
Sauerkraut 🔶
Seaweed
Spinach
Squash (crookneck, summer/ yellow)
Snap peas and snow peas
Swiss chard
Tomatoes (fresh and canned)
Tomato sauce 🔶
Tomato or vegetable juice 🔶
Turnips
Water chestnuts
Zucchini

PROTEIN

Meat, fish, poultry, cheese, eggs, and many types of plant-based foods give you protein along with some fat. Foods from this list are divided into 4 groups based on the amount of fat they contain. These groups are lean protein, medium-fat protein, high-fat protein, and plant-based protein. Most protein foods do not contain carbs, except for some plant-based protein foods. The chart below shows you what 1 protein choice (about 1 ounce) contains.

	CARBS (GRAMS)	PROTEIN (GRAMS)	FAT (GRAMS)	CALORIES
Lean protein	–	7	2	45
Medium-fat protein	–	7	5	75
High-fat protein	–	7	8	100
Plant-based protein	varies	7	varies	varies

Protein choices are often measured in 1-ounce portions. However, this is not the amount that most people would eat at a meal. For example, a breakfast sandwich with 1 ounce of cheese and 1 ounce of ham counts as 2 protein choices. Or a grilled chicken breast that is 3 ounces counts as 3 protein choices. Some snacks may also contain protein. Talk to your dietitian to learn more about how many protein choices are right for you each day.

Eating Plan Tips

- Whenever you can, choose lean cuts of meat and poultry because they have less saturated fat and cholesterol. You can also reduce the fat and cholesterol by trimming fat around the edges of meat and by removing the skin from poultry before eating.

- Many types of fish (such as herring, mackerel, salmon, sardines, halibut, trout, and tuna) contain healthy omega-3 fats, which may help reduce risk for heart disease. Choose fish (grilled or baked) 2 or more times each week.

- Read labels to find protein foods lower in fat. Aim for 5 grams of fat or fewer per protein choice (1-ounce serving size).

- Check labels of plant-based protein choices for hidden carbs. For example, meatless or vegetable burgers may contain carbs. Check the Nutrition Facts panel on the food label to see if the Total Carbohydrate in 1 serving is close to 15 grams. If it is close to 15 grams, count it as 1 carb choice and 1 protein choice.

- Processed meats, such as hot dogs and sausage, are often high in fat and sodium. Look for lower-fat and lower-sodium options and watch your portion size.

- Meat or fish that is breaded with cornmeal, flour, or dried bread crumbs contains carbs (count 3 tablespoons of these dry starches as 1 carb choice).

Lean Proteins

FOOD	AMOUNT
Beef: USDA Choice or Select grades, trimmed of fat: ground (90% or higher lean/10% or lower fat), roast (chuck, round, rump, sirloin), steak (cubed, flank, porterhouse, T-bone), tenderloin	1 oz
Beef jerky	½ oz
Cheeses with 3 grams of fat or less per oz	1 oz
Curd style cheeses: cottage-type (all kinds), ricotta (fat free or light)	¼ cup
Egg substitutes, plain	¼ cup
Egg whites	2
Fish: fresh or frozen, such as catfish, cod, flounder, haddock, halibut, orange roughy, tilapia, trout	1 oz
salmon, fresh or canned	1 oz
sardines, canned	2 small sardines
smoked herring or salmon (lox)	1 oz
tuna, fresh or canned in water or oil, drained	1 oz

Lean Proteins, continued

FOOD	AMOUNT
Game: buffalo, ostrich, rabbit, venison	1 oz
Goat: chop, leg, loin	1 oz
Hot dog with 3 grams of fat or less per oz (may contain carbs)	1 hot dog (1 ¾ oz)
Lamb: chop, leg, or roast	1 oz
Organ meats: heart, kidney, liver	1 oz
Pork, lean	
Canadian bacon	1 oz
ham	1 oz
rib or loin chop/roast, tenderloin	1 oz
Poultry, without skin: chicken, Cornish hen, domestic duck or goose (well-drained of fat), turkey; lean ground turkey or chicken	1 oz
Processed sandwich meats with 3 grams of fat or less per oz: chipped beef, thin-sliced deli meats, turkey ham, turkey pastrami	1 oz
Sausage with 3 grams of fat or less per oz	1 oz
Shellfish: clams, oysters, crab, lobster, scallops, shrimp	1 oz
Veal: cutlet (no breading), loin chop, roast	1 oz

Medium-Fat Proteins

FOOD	AMOUNT
Beef trimmed of visible fat: ground beef (85% or lower lean/15% or higher fat), corned beef, meatloaf, USDA prime cuts of beef (rib roast), short ribs, tongue	1 oz
Cheeses with 4 to 7 grams of fat per ounce: feta, mozzarella, pasteurized processed cheese spread, reduced-fat cheeses	1 oz
Cheese, ricotta (regular or part skim)	¼ cup (2 oz)
Egg	1 egg
Fish: any fried	1 oz
Lamb: ground, rib roast	1 oz
Pork: cutlet, ground, shoulder roast	1 oz
Poultry with skin: chicken, dove, pheasant, turkey, wild duck or goose, fried chicken	1 oz
Sausage with 4 to 7 grams of fat per oz	1 oz

High-Fat Proteins

These foods are higher in saturated fat, cholesterol, and calories and may raise blood cholesterol levels if eaten on a regular basis. Try to eat 3 or fewer servings from this group per week.

FOOD	SERVING SIZE
Bacon, pork	2 slices (1 oz each before cooking)
Bacon, turkey 🧡	3 slices (½ oz each before cooking)
Cheese, regular: American, blue-veined, brie, cheddar, hard goat, Monterey jack, parmesan, queso, and Swiss	1 oz
Hot dog: beef, pork, or combination ⚠️	1 hot dog (10 hot dogs per 1 lb-sized package)
Hot dog: turkey or chicken	1 hot dog (10 hot dogs per 1 lb-sized package)
Pork: sausage, spareribs	1 oz
Processed sandwich meats with 8 grams of fat or more per oz: bologna, hard salami, pastrami 🧡	1 oz
Sausage with 8 grams fat or more per oz: bratwurst, chorizo, Italian, knockwurst, Polish, smoked, summer 🧡	1 oz

Plant-Based Proteins

Because carb content varies among plant-based protein foods, check food labels for Total Carbohydrate amount (1 carb choice = about 15 grams of carbs).

FOOD	SERVING SIZE	CHOICES PER SERVING
"Bacon" strips, soy-based	2 strips (½ oz)	1 lean protein
Beans (black, garbanzo, kidney, lima, navy, pinto, white), cooked or canned, drained and rinsed ✅	½ cup	1 carb + 1 lean protein
"Beef" or "sausage" crumbles, meatless	1 oz	1 lean protein
"Chicken" nuggets, soy-based	2 nuggets (1½ oz)	½ carb + 1 medium-fat protein
Edamame, shelled ✅	½ cup	½ carb + 1 lean protein
Falafel (spiced chickpea and wheat patties)	3 patties (about 2 inches across)	1 carb + 1 high-fat protein
Hot dog, meatless	1 hot dog (1½ oz)	1 lean protein
Hummus ✅	⅓ cup	1 carb + 1 medium-fat protein
Lentils, cooked or canned, drained and rinsed ✅	½ cup	1 carb + 1 lean protein
Meatless burger, soy-based	3 oz	½ carb + 2 lean proteins

Plant-Based Proteins, continued

FOOD	SERVING SIZE	CHOICES PER SERVING
Meatless burger, vegetable- and starch-based ✅	1 patty (about 2½ oz)	½ carb + 1 lean protein
Meatless deli slices	1 oz	1 lean protein
Mycoprotein ("chicken" tenders), meatless	2 oz	½ carb + 1 lean protein
Nut spreads: almond butter, cashew butter, peanut butter, soy nut butter	1 Tbsp	1 high-fat protein
Peas (black-eyed and split peas), cooked or canned, drained and rinsed	½ cup	1 carb + 1 lean protein
Refried beans, canned ✅	½ cup	1 carb + 1 lean protein
"Sausage" breakfast-type patties, meatless	1 (1½ oz)	1 medium-fat protein
Soy nuts, unsalted	¾ oz	½ carb + 1 medium-fat protein
Tempeh, plain, unflavored	¼ cup (1½ oz)	1 medium-fat protein
Tofu	½ cup (4 oz)	1 medium-fat protein
Tofu, light	½ cup (4 oz)	1 lean protein

Beans, peas, and lentils are also found on the Starch list, page 27.

Nuts and nut butters in smaller amounts are found in the Fats list, page 52.

Canned beans, lentils, and peas can be high in sodium unless they are labeled *no salt added* or *low sodium*. Draining and rinsing canned beans, peas, and lentils reduces sodium by about 40%.

FATS

The fats on this list are divided into 3 groups, based on the main type of fat they contain:

- **Unsaturated fats** primarily come from vegetable sources and are healthier fats. There are 2 kinds of unsaturated fats:
  - Monounsaturated fats
  - Polyunsaturated fats (including omega-3 fats)
- **Saturated fats** primarily come from animal sources and are less healthy solid fats. **Trans fat,** a type of fat in some processed foods, is an unhealthy fat and should be avoided.

Eating Plan Tips

- When choosing fats, try to replace saturated fats with monounsaturated and polyunsaturated fat choices that are good sources of omega-3 fats. For example, use liquid fats, such as olive oil or canola oil instead of solid fats, such as butter, lard, shortening, or margarine for cooking or baking.
- Nuts and seeds are good sources of unsaturated fats and have small amounts of fiber and protein. Eat them in small amounts (see food lists) to reduce calories.
- Good sources of omega-3 fats include:
  - Fish, such as albacore tuna, halibut, herring, mackerel, salmon, sardines, and trout
  - Ground flaxseed and English walnuts

- Oils such as canola, soybean, flaxseed, and walnut
- 1 fat choice is based on a serving size that has 5 grams of total fat. Check the Nutrition Facts panel on food labels for actual amounts of fat in a serving. The label serving size may be different than the serving size used in this food list.

Trans fats

Trans fats are found naturally in some meat and dairy products. But most *trans* fats are made in a process that changes vegetable oils into semisolid fats. Avoid *trans* fats because they raise your risk for heart disease. *Trans* fats may be found in these types of processed foods:

- Solid vegetable shortening, stick margarines, and some tub margarines
- Crackers, candies, cookies, snack foods, fried foods, baked goods, coffee creamers, and other food items made with partially hydrogenated vegetable oils

To avoid *trans* fats in processed foods, look for products labeled "0 g *trans* fat" or "*trans* fat–free." You can also check the Nutrition Facts panel for the amount of *trans* fat. Keep in mind that some foods claiming to be *trans* fat–free may still contain a small amount of *trans* fat (less than ½ gram per serving). Check the ingredient list to be sure. If a "partially hydrogenated oil" or "hydrogenated oil" is listed, this means that a

Unsaturated Fats—Monounsaturated Fats

FOOD	SERVING SIZE
Almond milk (unsweetened)	1 cup
Avocado, medium	2 Tbsp (1 oz)
Nut butters (*trans* fat–free): almond butter, cashew butter, peanut butter (smooth or crunchy)	1½ tsp
Nuts	
almonds	6 nuts
Brazil	2 nuts
cashews	6 nuts
filberts (hazelnuts)	5 nuts
macadamia	3 nuts
mixed (50% peanuts)	6 nuts
peanuts	10 nuts
pecans	4 halves
pistachios	16 nuts
Oil: canola, olive, peanut	1 tsp
Olives	
black (ripe)	8
green, stuffed	10 large
Spread, plant stanol ester-type	

Unsaturated Fats—Monounsaturated Fats, continued

FOOD	SERVING SIZE
light	1 Tbsp
regular	2 tsp

Unsaturated Fats—Polyunsaturated Fats

FOOD	SERVING SIZE
Margarine	
lower-fat spread (30 to 50% vegetable oil, *trans* fat-free)	1 Tbsp
stick, tub (*trans* fat-free), or squeeze (*trans* fat-free)	1 tsp
Mayonnaise	
regular	1 tsp
reduced-fat	1 Tbsp
Mayonnaise-style salad dressing	
regular	2 tsp
reduced-fat	1 Tbsp
Nuts	
pignolia (pine nuts)	1 Tbsp
walnuts, English	4 halves
Oil: corn, cottonseed, flaxseed, grape seed, safflower, soybean, sunflower	1 tsp
Salad dressing	

Unsaturated Fats—Polyunsaturated Fats, continued

FOOD	SERVING SIZE
regular	1 Tbsp
reduced-fat (may contain carbs)	2 Tbsp
Seeds	
flaxseed, ground	1½ Tbsp
pumpkin, sesame, sunflower	1 Tbsp
Tahini or sesame paste	2 tsp

Saturated Fats

FOOD	SERVING SIZE
Bacon, cooked, regular or turkey	1 slice
Butter	
reduced-fat	1 Tbsp
stick	1 tsp
whipped	2 tsp
Butter blends made with oil	
reduced-fat or light	1 Tbsp
regular	1½ tsp
Chitterlings, boiled (chitlins)	2 Tbsp (½ oz)
Coconut, sweetened, shredded	2 Tbsp
Coconut milk (canned, thick)	
regular	1½ Tbsp
light	⅓ cup

Saturated Fats, continued

FOOD	SERVING SIZE
Coconut milk beverage (thin), unsweetened	1 cup
Cream	
half and half	2 Tbsp
heavy	1 Tbsp
light	1½ Tbsp
whipped	2 Tbsp
Cream cheese	
reduced-fat	1½ Tbsp (¾ oz)
regular	1 Tbsp (½ oz)
Lard	1 tsp
Oil: coconut, palm, palm kernel	1 tsp
Salt pork	¼ oz
Shortening, solid	1 tsp
Sour cream	
reduced-fat or light	3 Tbsp
regular	2 Tbsp

COMBINATION FOODS

Many of the foods we eat, such as casseroles, sandwiches, frozen meals, and fast foods, have a lot of different ingredients. These "combination" foods do not fit into any single Choice list. Combination foods may be made at home, away from home, or delivered to your home. This list will help you learn how these foods fit into your eating plan. Ask your dietitian about nutrition information for other combination foods you would like to eat, including your own recipes.

Main Dishes/Entrées

FOOD	SERVING SIZE	CHOICES PER SERVING
Bowl, vegetarian (vegetable, tofu, rice) ✅ 🥫	8–10 oz	3 carbs + 1 lean protein + 1 fat
Bowl with chicken or beef and rice 🥫	8–10 oz	2 carbs + 2 lean proteins + 1 fat
Chicken		
breast, breaded and fried* 🥫	1 (about 7 oz)	1 carb + 6 medium-fat proteins
drumstick, breaded and fried*	1 (about 2½ oz)	½ carb + 2 medium-fat proteins

FOOD	SERVING SIZE	CHOICES PER SERVING
nuggets or tenders 🔶	6 (about 3½ oz)	1 carb + 2 medium-fat proteins + 1 fat
thigh, breaded and fried* 🔶	1 (about 5 oz)	1 carb + 3 medium-fat proteins + 2 fats
wing, breaded and fried*	1 wing (about 2 oz)	½ carb + 2 medium-fat proteins
Casserole-type entrees (tuna noodle, lasagna, spaghetti with meatballs, chili with beans, macaroni and cheese) 🔶	1 cup (8 oz)	2 carbs + 2 medium-fat proteins
Pizza		
cheese/vegetarian, thin crust 🔶	¼ of a 12-inch pizza (4½–5 oz)	2 carbs + 2 medium-fat proteins
meat topping, thin crust 🔶	¼ of a 12-inch pizza (5 oz)	2 carbs + 2 medium-fat proteins + 1½ fats
cheese, meat, and vegetable, regular crust 🔶	⅛ of a 14-inch pizza (about 5 oz)	2½ carbs + 2 high-fat proteins

Main Dishes/Entrées, continued

FOOD	SERVING SIZE	CHOICES PER SERVING
Pot pie (meat or vegetarian)	1 pot pie (7 oz)	3 carbs + 1 lean protein + 3 fats
Stews (beef/other meats and vegetables)	1 cup (8 oz)	1 carb + 1 medium-fat protein + 0 to 3 fats
Salad, main dish (grilled chicken-type, no dressing or croutons)	1 salad (about 11 ½ oz)	1 carb + 4 lean proteins
Tuna salad or chicken salad	½ cup (3 ½ oz)	½ carb +2 lean proteins + 1 fat

*Definition and weight refer to food with bone, skin, and breading.

Asian

FOOD	SERVING SIZE	CHOICES PER SERVING
Beef/chicken/shrimp with vegetables in sauce 🔶	1 cup (about 6 oz)	1 carb + 2 lean proteins + 1 fat
Egg roll, meat	1 egg roll (about 3 oz)	1½ carbs + 1 lean protein + 1½ fats
Fried rice, meatless	1 cup	2½ carbs + 2 fats
Brown rice, steamed (rice cooker)	1 cup	3 carbs
Hot and sour soup 🔶	1 cup	½ carb + ½ fat
Meat and sweet sauce 🔶	1 cup (about 6 oz)	3½ carbs + 3 medium-fat proteins + 3 fats
Noodles and vegetables in sauce (chow mein, lo mein) 🔶	1 cup	2 carbs + 2 fats
Pad Thai noodles, with chicken 🔶	1 cup	3 carbs + 2 lean proteins + 2 fats
Pho: beef broth, rice noodles, and meat 🔶	3 cups	4 carbs + 2 medium-fat proteins + 1 fat
Sushi: fish and rice (without soy sauce)	2 pieces	1 carb + 1 lean protein + 1 fat
California rolls (without soy sauce)	2 pieces	1 carb + 1 fat
Tikka masala with chicken 🔶	1 cup	1 carb + 3 lean proteins + 2 fats

Mexican

FOOD	SERVING SIZE	CHOICES PER SERVING
Burrito with beans and cheese ✅ 🧂	1 small burrito (about 6 oz)	3½ carbs + 1 medium-fat protein + 1 fat
Burrito with beans and beef ✅ 🧂	1 small burrito (about 5 oz)	3 carbs + 1 lean protein + 2 fats
Nachos with cheese 🧂	1 small order (about 8 nachos)	2½ carbs + 1 high-fat protein + 2 fats
Quesadilla, cheese only 🧂	1 small order (about 5 oz)	2½ carbs + 3 high-fat proteins
Taco, crisp, with meat and cheese 🧂	1 small taco (about 3 oz)	1 carb + 1 medium-fat protein + 1½ fats
Taco salad with chicken and tortilla bowl ✅ 🧂	1 salad (1 lb, including tortilla bowl)	3½ carbs + 4 medium-fat proteins + 3 fats
Tostada with beans and cheese ✅ 🧂	1 small tostada (about 5 oz)	2 carbs + 1 high-fat protein

Sandwiches

FOOD	SERVING SIZE	CHOICES PER SERVING
Breakfast Sandwiches		
breakfast burrito with sausage, egg, cheese 🔸	1 small burrito (about 4 oz)	1½ carbs + 2 high-fat proteins
egg, cheese, meat on an English muffin 🔸	1 sandwich	2 carbs + 3 medium-fat proteins + ½ fat
egg, cheese, meat on a biscuit or croissant 🔸	1 sandwich	2 carbs + 3 medium-fat proteins + 2 fats
Chicken Sandwiches		
grilled with bun, lettuce, tomatoes, spread 🔸	1 sandwich (about 7½ oz)	3 carbs + 4 lean proteins
crispy, with bun, lettuce, tomatoes, spread 🔸	1 sandwich (about 6 oz)	3 carbs + 2 lean proteins + 3½ fats
pocket sandwich 🔸	1 sandwich (4½ oz)	3 carbs + 1 lean protein + 1 to 2 fats
Fish Sandwich, breaded, with bun, tartar sauce, cheese, lettuce, and tomato 🔸	1 sandwich (5 oz)	2½ carbs + 2 medium-fat proteins + 1½ fats

Sandwiches, continued

FOOD	SERVING SIZE	CHOICES PER SERVING
Hamburger		
regular with bun and condiments (ketchup, mustard, onion, pickle) 🥤	1 small burger (about 3½ oz)	2 carbs + 1 medium-fat protein + 1 fat
4-oz meat with cheese, bun, and condiments (ketchup, mustard, onion, pickle) 🥤	1 burger (about 8½ oz)	3 carbs + 4 medium-fat proteins + 2½ fats
Hot dog with bun, plain 🥤	1 hot dog (about 3½ oz)	1½ carbs + 1 high-fat protein + 2 fats
Submarine sandwich (no cheese or sauce)		
less than 6 grams fat 🥤	6-inch sub	3 carbs + 2 lean proteins
regular	6-inch sub	3 carbs + 2 lean proteins + 1 fat
Wrap, grilled chicken, vegetables, cheese, and spread	1 small wrap (about 4 to 5 oz)	2 carbs + 2 lean proteins + 1½ fats

Side Dishes

FOOD	SERVING SIZE	CHOICES PER SERVING
Coleslaw, creamy	½ cup	1 carb + 1 ½ fats
Macaroni/pasta salad 🥕	½ cup	2 carbs + 3 fats
Potato salad 🥕	½ cup	1½ to 2 carbs + 1 or 2 fats
French fries, restaurant (fast food) style 🥕		
1 small order	about 3½ oz	2½ carbs + 2 fats
1 medium order	about 5 oz	3½ carbs + 3 fats
1 large order	about 6 oz	4½ carbs + 4 fats
Onion rings 🥕	1 serving (8 to 9 rings, about 4 oz)	3½ carbs + 4 fats

Soups

FOOD	SERVING SIZE	CHOICES PER SERVING
Bean, lentil, or split pea soup ✓ 🍶	1 cup (8 oz)	2 carbs + 1 lean protein
Chowder (made with milk) 🍶	1 cup (8 oz)	1 carb + 1 lean protein + 1½ fats
Cream soup (made with water) 🍶	1 cup (8 oz)	1 carb + 1 fat
Miso soup 🍶	1 cup (8 oz)	½ carb + 1 lean protein
Ramen noodle soup 🍶	1 cup (8 oz)	2 carbs + 2 fats
Rice soup/porridge (congee) 🍶	1 cup (8 oz)	1 carb
Tomato soup (made with water), borscht 🍶	1 cup (8 oz)	1 carb
Vegetable beef, chicken noodle, or other broth-type soup (including "healthy"-type soups, such as those lower in sodium and/or fat) 🍶	1 cup (8 oz)	1 carb + 1 lean protein

Tips for Eating Out

- Plan ahead. Make a list of fast food places and restaurants near you that offer more healthy choices.

- Ask questions before you place your order:

- How is the item prepared? Can you substitute items?

- Ask for more vegetables whenever you can.

- Choose whole-grain breads and brown rice, when available.

- Avoid items that are "jumbo," "giant," "deluxe," or "super-sized."

- Watch out for hidden extra calories, such as croutons, bacon, or cheese.

- Ask for salad dressings, sour cream, and butter on the side so you can decide how much to use.

- Don't forget that many drinks contain calories and carbs.

- Look for nutrition information online for many restaurants, including calories, carbs, and fats, or ask for nutrition information before you place your order.

SWEETS, DESSERTS, AND OTHER CARBOHYDRATES

The American Diabetes Association and the Academy of Nutrition and Dietetics nutrition guidelines state that people with diabetes can enjoy sugar and foods containing sugar in small amounts, if desired. While foods on this list can and do affect your blood glucose, they do not cause diabetes. These foods can be part of an eating plan in small amounts instead of other carb foods. Foods on this list have added sugars and fat, and often little or no nutrients like vitamins, minerals, and fiber. Talk to your dietitian about how to fit these foods in your eating plan if you choose to eat them.

Eating Plan Tips

- Many of the foods on the **Sweets, Desserts, and Other Carbohydrates** list contain more than a single choice of carbs. Some will also count as 1 or more fat choices.

- The serving sizes for these foods are small because of their high carbs and fat content. Read the Nutrition Facts panel on the food label to find the serving size and nutrient information. Remember: The label serving size may be different from the serving size used in this food list.

- Many sugar-free, fat-free, or reduced-fat products are made with ingredients that contain carbs. These types of food often have the same amount of carbs as the regular foods they are replacing.

Beverages, Soda, and Sports Drinks

FOOD	SERVING SIZE	CHOICES PER SERVING
Energy drink	1 can (about 8 fl oz)	2 carbs
Fruit drink or lemonade	1 cup (8 fl oz)	2 carbs
Hot chocolate, regular	1 envelope (2 Tbsp or ¾ oz) added to 8 fl oz water, or added to 8 fl oz milk	1 carb 2 carbs
Soft drink (soda), regular	1 can (12 fl oz)	2½ carbs
Sports drink (fluid replacement type)	1 cup (8 fl oz)	1 carb

Brownies, Cake, Cookies, Gelatin, Pie, and Pudding

FOOD	SERVING SIZE	CHOICES PER SERVING
Biscotti	1 oz	1 carb + 1 fat
Brownie, small, unfrosted	1¼-inch square, ⅞-inch high (about 1 oz)	1 carb + 1 fat
Cake		
angel food, unfrosted	¹⁄₁₂ of cake (about 2 oz)	2 carbs

Brownies, Cake, Cookies, Gelatin, Pie, and Pudding, continued

FOOD	SERVING SIZE	CHOICES PER SERVING
frosted	2-inch square (about 2 oz)	2 carbs + 1 fat
unfrosted	2-inch square (about 1 oz)	1 carb + 1 fat
gluten-free, unfrosted	1/10 of cake (about 1 oz)	2½ carbs
Cookies		
100-calorie pack	1 oz	1 carb + ½ fat
chocolate chip cookies	2 small, 2¼ inches across	1 carb + 2 fats
gluten-free chocolate chip cookies	2 small	1 carb + 1 fat
gingersnaps	3 small, 1½ inches across	1 carb
large cookie	1 cookie, 6 inches across (about 3 oz)	4 carbs + 3 fats
sandwich cookies with creme filling	2 small (about ⅔ oz)	1 carb + 1 fat
sugar-free cookies	1 large or 3 small (¾ to 1 oz)	1 carb + 1 to 2 fats
vanilla wafer	5 cookies	1 carb + 1 fat

FOOD	SERVING SIZE	CHOICES PER SERVING
Cupcake, frosted	1 small (about 1¾ oz)	2 carbs + 1 to 1½ fats
Flan	½ cup	2½ carbs + 1 fat
Fruit cobbler	½ cup (3½ oz)	3 carbs + 1 fat
Gelatin, regular	½ cup	1 carb
Pie		
commercially prepared fruit, 2 crusts	⅙ of 8-inch pie	3 carbs + 2 fats
pumpkin or custard	⅛ of 8-inch pie	1½ carbs + 1½ fats
Pudding		
regular (made with reduced-fat milk)	½ cup	2 carbs
sugar-free or sugar- and fat-free (made with fat-free milk)	½ cup	1 carb

Candy, Spreads, Sweets, Sweeteners, Syrups, and Toppings

FOOD	SERVING SIZE	CHOICES PER SERVING
Agave, syrup	1 Tbsp	1 carb
Blended sweeteners	1½ Tbsp	1 carb
Candy, chocolate, dark or milk	1 oz	1 carb + 2 fats
Candy, hard	3 pieces	1 carb
Chocolate "kisses"	5 pieces	1 carb + 1 fat
Coffee creamer, nondairy type		
dry, flavored	4 tsp	½ carb + ½ fat
liquid, flavored	2 Tbsp	1 carb
Fruit snacks, chewy (puréed fruit concentrate)	1 roll (¾ oz)	1 carb
Fruit spreads, 100% fruit	1½ Tbsp	1 carb
Honey	1 Tbsp	1 carb
Jam or jelly, regular	1 Tbsp	1 carb
Sugar (white granular, molasses, brown sugar packed)	1 Tbsp	1 carb
Syrup		
chocolate	2 Tbsp	2 carbs
light (pancake type)	2 Tbsp	1 carb
regular (pancake type)	1 Tbsp	1 carb

Sugar Alcohols

Sugar alcohols are a type of carbohydrate that provides a sweet taste with fewer calories per gram than regular sugar (sucrose). They can be used in place of sugar, often along with sugar substitutes. Products that may contain sugar alcohols include sugar-free candies, gum, dairy, desserts, and baked goods.

- To find out if a product contains sugar alcohols, check the label. Sugar alcohol is sometimes listed below sugars on the Nutrition Facts panel on a food label. You can also check the ingredients list to see what type is in your food, such as erythritol, glycerol, hydrogenated starch hydrolysate, isomalt, lactitol, maltitol, mannitol, sorbitol, and xylitol.

- Sugar alcohols can cause your blood glucose to be lower after a meal because the body does not fully digest them. Foods that have sugar alcohols can be labeled as "sugar-free," but this doesn't mean they are carb-free or calorie-free.

- In some people, sugar alcohols can cause bloating, gas, or diarrhea. Foods that contain the sugar alcohols sorbitol or mannitol must include a warning on their label that states "excess consumption may have a laxative effect."

Donuts, Muffins, Pastries, and Sweet Breads

FOOD	SERVING SIZE	CHOICES PER SERVING
Banana nut bread	1-inch slice (2 oz)	2 carbs + 1 fat
Donut		
cake, plain	1 medium donut (1½ oz)	1½ carbs + 2 fats
hole	2 holes (1 oz)	1 carb + 1 fat
yeast type, glazed	1 donut, 3¾ inches across (2 oz)	2 carbs + 2 fats
Muffin		
regular	1 muffin (4 oz)	4 carbs + 2½ fats
lower fat	1 muffin (4 oz)	4 carbs + ½ fat
gluten-free, blueberry	1 muffin (3 oz)	3 carbs + 2 fats
Scone	1 scone (4 oz)	4 carbs + 3 fats
Sweet roll or Danish	1 pastry (2½ oz)	2½ carbs + 2 fats

Frozen Bars, Frozen Desserts, Frozen Yogurt, and Ice Cream

FOOD	SERVING SIZE	CHOICES PER SERVING
Frozen pops	1	½ carb
Fruit juice bars, frozen, 100% juice	1 bar (3 oz)	1 carb
Ice cream		
fat-free	½ cup	1½ carbs
light	½ cup	1 carb + 1 fat
no sugar added	½ cup	1 carb + 1 fat
dairy-free, vegan (almond milk)	½ cup	1 carb + 2 fats
regular	½ cup	1 carb + 2 fats
Sherbet, sorbet	½ cup	2 carbs
Yogurt, frozen		
fat-free	⅓ cup	1 carb
regular	½ cup	1 carb + 0 to 1 fat
Greek, lower fat or fat-free	½ cup	1½ carbs

SNACKS AND EXTRAS

Snacks and extras can be a part of a healthy eating plan, and they can include many foods. If weight loss is your goal, eating a snack when you are not hungry can add extra calories that will make it harder to lose weight. There is no set number of snacks for all people with diabetes. However, based on your personal diabetes self-care and eating plan, you may include a snack if:

- Your meal will be later than usual
- You are more active than usual
- You take a diabetes medicine that causes your blood glucose level to get too low
- You are hungry

Carbohydrate Snacks

In the amounts listed below, these snacks are equal to 1 carb choice or 15 grams of carbs. The amounts are common snack-size portions.

Fruit

1 small fresh fruit (about 2 ½ inches in diameter)
½ cup unsweetened canned fruit
½ cup unsweetened applesauce
½ cup fresh fruit salad
¼ cup dried fruit or 2 tablespoons raisins

Crunchy

3 cups light or air-popped popcorn
2 rice or popcorn cakes (4 inches across)
20 small pretzels (¾ ounce total)

3 graham crackers (2½-inch square)
2 breadsticks, crisp (4 inches long and ½ inch wide)
4 to 6 whole-wheat crackers
20 oyster crackers
15 to 20 snack chips (¾ ounce total; baked tortilla, potato, or pita chips)

Sweets

½ cup frozen yogurt, ice milk, or light ice cream
½ cup sugar-free pudding
8 animal crackers
5 vanilla wafers
1 frozen fruit pop
1 or 2 small cookies

Protein Snacks

The foods listed below count as about 1 protein choice or 7 grams of protein.

- 1 ounce of lean meat, turkey, or chicken
- 1 ounce of cheese (low-fat types with less than 5 grams of fat per ounce, such as mozzarella or feta)
- ¼ cup nuts, such as almonds, walnuts, or peanuts
- ¼ cup cottage cheese (part-skim or low-fat)
- 2 tablespoons peanut butter
- 1 hard-boiled egg

Very Low-Calorie and Low-Carb Snacks

The foods listed below have 20 calories or fewer, or 5 grams of carbs or fewer. An asterisk (*) after the food means it is high in sodium (salt). With the exception of the nonstarchy vegetables, the portion size of these snacks is very small.

- **Nonstarchy Vegetables** listed on pages 40–41; for example, 1 cup raw vegetables such as baby carrots, celery, or sugar snap peas, 3 cups salad greens, or 1 large unsweetened pickle.*

- **Fruits** food choices listed foods on pages 29–32; for example, ¼ cup blueberries or blackberries, ⅓ cup melon, 6 grapes, or 2 teaspoons dried fruits.

- **Starch** food choices listed on pages 26–27; for example, 2 animal crackers, 1 ½ saltine-type crackers, ¾ cup no-fat added popcorn, or ½ regular-sized rice or popcorn cake.

- **Fats** food choices listed on pages 52–46; for example, 8 pistachios, 3 almonds, 4 black olives, or 1 ½ teaspoons sunflower seeds.

- **Lean Protein** food choices listed on pages 44–45; for example, ½-ounce slice of fat-free cheese or ½ ounce of lean cooked meat.

- Other choices:
  - Fat-free bouillon or broth*
  - Diet or sugar-free gelatin
  - Diet or sugar-free soda pop, seltzer water, or club soda
  - Coffee or tea
  - Sugar-free drink mixes

Condiments and Sauces

FOOD	SERVING SIZE	CHOICES PER SERVING
Barbecue sauce	3 Tbsp	1 carb
Cranberry sauce, jellied	¼ cup	1½ carbs
Curry sauce	1 oz	1 carb + 1 fat
Gravy, canned or bottled	½ cup	½ carb + ½ fat
Hoisin sauce	1 Tbsp	½ carb
Hot chile sauce	1 Tbsp	½ carb
Ketchup	3 Tbsp	1 carb
Plum sauce	1 Tbsp	½ carb
Salad dressing, fat-free, cream-based	3 Tbsp	1 carb
Sweet and sour sauce	3 Tbsp	1 carb

NOTE: Many other condiments are very low in calories and carbs when eaten in small amounts. Check the Fats list on pages 53–55 for more condiments.

Sugar Substitutes

Sugar substitutes, alternatives, or replacements that are approved by the Food and Drug Administration (FDA) are safe to use. Each sweetener is tested for safety before it can be sold. Common types include the following:

- Aspartame, neotame (blue packet)
- Monk fruit (orange packet)
- Saccharin (pink packet)
- Stevia (green packet) (Stevia leaf and crude stevia extracts are not FDA-approved.)
- Sucralose (yellow packet)

If you choose foods made with sugar substitutes, check the label for other ingredients that contain calories, such as carbs, protein, and fats. Eating sugar substitutes is a personal choice. If you have questions on how they fit in your eating plan, talk with your dietitian.

ALCOHOL

Drinks that contain alcohol have different amounts of alcohol and carbs in them. Alcohol is not a nutrient, but alcohol has calories.

Eating Plan Tips

- If you take insulin or oral medications that cause a release of insulin from your pancreas, such as glipizide, glyburide or glimepiride, you risk having low blood glucose when you drink alcohol. Drinking alcohol on an empty stomach will increase this risk, so be sure you eat a meal when drinking alcohol.

- Alcohol alone does not have much effect on your blood glucose. What you mix with the alcohol could affect your blood glucose. Soda pop, juice, tonic, energy drinks, premade mixes (like margarita, daiquiri, or cosmopolitan mixes) often contain a lot of sugar.

- For less sugar and fewer calories, try mixing your drink with seltzer water, diet soda, diet tonic, light or no-sugar juices, light lemonade, sugar-free drink mixes, or sugar-free syrups.

- A serving or "drink" is considered 12 fluid ounces of beer, 5 fluid ounces of wine, or 1½ fluid ounces of hard alcohol like vodka, whiskey, rum, etc. A "shot" of alcohol can vary, but is usually 1½ fluid ounces.

- People with diabetes have the same guidelines for drinking alcohol as those without diabetes. For women who choose to drink, health professionals suggest limiting alcohol to 1 drink or less per day, and no alcoholic drinks for pregnant women. The suggested amount for men who choose to drink is no more than 2 drinks per day.

Alcoholic Beverages

ALCOHOLIC BEVERAGE	SERVING SIZE	CALORIES	CARB CHOICES (PER SERVING)
Beer			
light (4.2% abv)	12 fl oz	100	½
regular (~5% abv)	12 fl oz	150	1
dark (more than 5% abv)	12 fl oz	175	1 to 1½
Distilled spirits (80 or 86 proof): vodka, rum, gin, whiskey, tequila, cognac	1½ fl oz	100	0
Liqueurs			
coffee (53 proof)	1½ fl oz	150	1
Irish cream	1 fl oz	100	½ (+ 1 fat choice)
herbal liqueur (Jägermeister, 70 proof)	1 fl oz	100	1

Alcoholic Beverages, continued

ALCOHOLIC BEVERAGE	SERVING SIZE	CALORIES	CARB CHOICES (PER SERVING)
Sake (~15% abv)	3 fl oz	115	0
Wine			
Champagne	4 fl oz	80	0
dessert (sherry)	3 ½ fl oz	150	1
red, rosé, or white (10% abv)	5 fl oz	100 to 125	0

NOTE: The abbreviation "% abv" refers to the percentage of alcohol by volume.

READING FOOD LABELS

The Nutrition Facts panel and ingredients list on a food label can help you with your food choices. For more help using the information on food labels, ask your dietitian.

Check the Serving Size. Calorie and nutrient information on the label is for 1 serving of this size. NOTE: This amount is not always the same size as 1 choice listed in this booklet.

Look at Calories per serving. Use the calories listed to compare similar products (check that serving size is the same).

Look at the grams of Total Fat in 1 serving (1 fat choice has 5 grams of fat).

To help lower your risk of heart disease, try to

Nutrition Facts

8 servings per container
Serving size   2/3 cup (55g)

Amount per serving
Calories   230

	% Daily Value*
Total Fat 8g	10%
Saturated Fat 1g	5%
Trans Fat 0g	
Cholesterol 0mg	0%
Sodium 160mg	7%
Total Carbohydrate 37g	13%
Dietary Fiber 4g	14%
Total Sugars 12g	
Includes 10g Added Sugars	20%
Protein 3g	
Vitamin D 2mcg	10%
Calcium 260mg	20%
Iron 8mg	45%
Potassium 235mg	6%

* The % Daily Value (DV) tells you how much a nutrient in a serving of food contributes to a daily diet. 2,000 calories a day is used for general nutrition advice.

Ingredients: water, tomato purée (water, tomato paste), seasoned beef crumbles (beef, salt, spice extracts), diced tomatoes in tomato juice, red kidney beans, kidney beans. Contains less than 2% of the following ingredients: concentrate (caramel color added), jalapeno peppers, salt, dehydrated onions, **sugar**, dehydrated garlic, paprika, red pepper, soybean oil, soy lecithin, mono and diglycerides, mixed tocopherols, ascorbic acid, flavoring.

choose foods that are low in saturated fats, *trans* fats, and cholesterol.

Check the grams of Total Carbohydrate. This is the total amount of starches, natural and added sugars, sugar alcohols, and dietary fiber in a food. To figure out how many carb choices are in 1 serving, divide the Total Carbohydrate amount by 15 (1 carb choice has 15 grams of carbs).

Look for foods that have Dietary Fiber. A good source of fiber is about 3 grams of fiber per serving and an excellent source has at least 5 grams or more per serving.

Choose foods that are lower in Added Sugars. Total sugars include sugars that are naturally in foods (such as fruit and dairy products) and sugars that are added to foods. Added sugars tell you how much of the Total Carbohydrate amount comes from sugars added to the food. Every 4 grams of sugar is equal to 1 teaspoon. **The ingredient list** provides information about the types of sugars added to food.

INDEX

veal, 45

vegetable. *See also under specific type*
   canned/frozen, 39
   eating out, 65
   juice, 41
   nonstarchy, 14–15, 38–41, 76
   starchy, 15, 19–20, 25
vegetable soup with meat, 64
vegetarian bowl, 56
very low-calorie snack, 75–76
vitamin D, 34

W

waffle, 122
walking, 4–5
water chestnut, 41
watermelon, 32
weight, 3–4
weight loss, 3, 74
wheat germ, 23
whole grain, 19–20, 24, 65
whole-wheat cracker, 75

wine, 81
wrap, 62

Y

yam, 25
yogurt, 34, 36–37
yogurt, frozen, 73, 75

Z

zucchini, 41

Eating Plan For: _____ Date: _____

RDN: _____ Contact: _____

Daily Amounts:

Carbohydrate _____ choices   Proteins _____ choices   Fats _____ choices

Total Calories

	STARCH	FRUIT	MILK AND MILK SUBSTITUTES	NONSTARCHY VEGETABLES	TOTAL CARBOHYDRATE (CHOICES) (GRAMS)		PROTEIN	FAT	MENU IDEAS
BREAKFAST Time:									
LUNCH Time:									
DINNER Time:									
SNACKS* Time: Time:									

The Diabetes Plate is a great way to estimate your portions and create a meal with a healthy balance of vegetables, protein, and carbs. All you need is a plate that is 9 inches across. Now that you have the right plate, it's time to fill it!

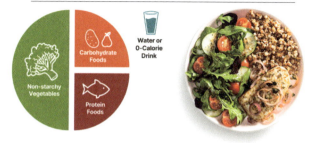

Step 1

Fill one half of your plate with nonstarchy vegetables. Examples can be found on pages 40–41 of this book. Nonstarchy vegetables have fewer carbs and calories compared to starchy vegetables (such as potatoes, corn, and peas), and many also provide fiber.

Step 2

Fill one quarter of your plate with protein foods. For animal proteins, lean proteins such as chicken, turkey, and fish are usually best as they contain less saturated fat, which can increase your risk of heart disease.

Plant-based protein sources include beans, lentils, hummus, tofu, and tempeh. Keep in mind that some, like beans and legumes, are also high in carbohydrate.

Step 3

Fill the last quarter of your plate with carbohydrate foods. Foods that are higher in carbs include whole grains, starchy vegetables, beans and legumes, fruit, yogurt, and milk. These foods have the largest effect on blood glucose.

Limiting your portion of carbohydrate foods to one-quarter of your plate can help keep blood glucose from rising too high after meals.